POCKET
DETOX

Ordering
Trade bookstores in the U.S. and Canada please contact:
Publishers Group West
1700 Fourth Street, Berkeley CA 94710
Phone: (800) 788-3123   Fax: (800) 351-5073

For bulk orders please contact:
Special Sales
Hunter House Inc., PO Box 2914, Alameda CA 94501-0914
Phone: (510) 899-5041   Fax: (510) 865-4295
E-mail: sales@hunterhouse.com

Individuals can order by calling **(800) 266-5592**
or from our website at **www.hunterhouse.com**

POCKET
DETOX

CATHERINE PROCTOR

Library of Congress Cataloging-in-Publication Data
Proctor, Catherine.
Pocket detox / Catherine Proctor. — [1st] U.S. ed.
p. cm.
Originally published: Paddington, N.S.W. : Jane Curry Pub., 2006.
Includes index.
ISBN 978-0-89793-642-2 (pbk.)
1. Detoxification (Health) 2. Lifestyles. I. Title.
RA784.5.P76 2012
613.2—dc23   2012019235

Project Credits

Cover Design: Jinni Fontana	Rights Coordinator:
Book Production: John McKercher	Candace Groskreutz
Copy Editor: Heather Wilcox	Customer Service Manager:
Proofreader: Lori Cavanaugh	Christina Sverdrup
Indexer: Candace Hyatt	Order Fulfillment: Washul Lakdhon
Managing Editor: Alexandra Mummery	Administrator: Theresa Nelson
Acquisitions Assistant: Elana Fiske	Computer Support:
Special Sales Manager: Judy Hardin	Peter Eichelberger
Publisher: Kiran S. Rana	

Printed and bound by Bang Printing, Brainerd, Minnesota
Manufactured in the United States of America

9 8 7 6 5 4 3 2 1   First Edition   12 13 14 15 16

Contents

Introduction

Contrary to popular belief, detox living is not about following fad diets or losing weight (although weight loss is a great side effect of detoxing). Detoxing simply focuses on removing toxins from your body, mind, and environment to enable you to function at your full potential.

Detoxing can help you increase your energy levels, feel more relaxed, and achieve physical well-being. It can also lead to better overall health with some amazing side effects, such as losing weight and kicking addictions.

You do not have to purchase a lot of vitamin supplements, drink foul-tasting concoctions, or spend a fortune at an exclusive health farm to detox. With the help of *Pocket Detox*, you can safely detox by modifying your diet and lifestyle.

Pocket Detox also provides tips on removing toxins from your home, cleansing your environment, and learning relaxation techniques to help manage stress.

Ultimately, you decide how to use *Pocket Detox*. You can use it as a guide to help you change your overall lifestyle and eating habits, or you may want to refer to it to do a weekend or weeklong detox whenever you start to feel rundown and overloaded.

Either way, *Pocket Detox* will help you take control of your health and eat your way to a happier, healthier, and more-energized lifestyle.

What Are Toxins?

Toxins are basically poisonous by-products of the modern lifestyle. Detoxing is quite simply a way of removing toxins from your diet, body, and home. Because toxins are already slowly clogging up your environment, you need to do what you can to remove these toxins from your life.

So what are you doing to invite these toxins into your body? Here are some of the most common causes:

- highly processed food
- smoking
- alcohol
- caffeine
- stress

And not getting enough of the following:

- sleep
- water
- exercise
- fresh, unprocessed foods
- relaxation

How Your Body Works

Your body is a highly sophisticated machine that takes in food, fluids, and air to survive. Your internal organs process these elements to absorb the nutrients that you need to survive. They then eliminate the waste and by-products.

Although the human body is very adaptable and works to maintain an internal balance, if you overload it with toxins, it will not be able to function properly, and it will let you know that it needs help.

If you think of your body as a high-performance vehicle, you can quite easily see why it sometimes needs a tune-up:

- **Eating the wrong sorts of food** is like filling the tank with the wrong sort of gasoline. The result is sluggish, below-par performance.

- **Not exercising** is like not driving a car on a regular basis. The results are a flat battery and a car that cannot run at top speed.

- **Experiencing too much stress and no time-out** is like missing your car's regular service appointment. The results are breakdowns and a shorter life.

- Consuming **too much caffeine and alcohol** is like putting pollutants into the car's engine. The results are bad performance and the possibility of destroying your car's engine.

Other Types of Toxins

Toxins are not just present in the things that your body eats and drinks—they also need to be removed from your lifestyle, home, and personal life.

▌*Stress*

The brain is the most important organ in your body, and your emotional health is as important as your physical health. Stress often manifests itself in physical symptoms, such as loss of appetite, skin rashes, and sleep problems.

Learning to cope with and reduce stress is vital for your physical and emotional well-being. Although some causes of stress can be minimized, it is totally unrealistic to believe that you can remove all causes of stress from your life. Exercise, relaxation techniques, and stress management can all help you cope with the inevitable stress that is part of modern living.

▌*Environment*

Many toxins are present in your environment that you are not even aware of, including some that you have no control over, such as pollution.

What you can do to make a difference is minimize your own impact on the environment and reduce the toxin levels in your own home. Main causes of toxins in your home include the cleaning products you use and the materials chosen for the construction of your home. By simply choosing green cleaning methods, you can save money and reduce the amount of toxins in your environment.

What Are the Signs That Your Body Needs Help?

If you listen to your body, you will know when it needs help. Some of the common signs that your body is losing the battle against toxins include:

- allergies
- bad breath
- bloating
- coffee cravings
- headaches
- irritable bowel syndrome
- lethargy
- poor skin condition
- red, sore eyes
- reflux and indigestion
- sleep problems
- sugar cravings

These symptoms are all signs that something is wrong and that your body is not functioning at its full potential. Learn to listen to your body, and you will recognize when it is out of balance and needs help before you develop major health problems.

Take the Detox Quiz 2

Before you start to detox, take the detox quiz to determine your current state of health. The purpose of this quiz is to help you become more aware of the particular areas of your lifestyle that need some extra attention.

Are You Getting Enough Water?

Water is vital for your body's proper functioning. Your body consists of 80 percent water, so it is very important to maintain those water levels. If you do not drink enough water, your body will remove fluids from your bowels. This process slows down the removal of intestinal waste, causing toxins to be reabsorbed through the intestinal wall.

How many glasses of water do you drink each day?

    A fewer than three

    B three to six

    C six or more

How often do you drink carbonated cola drinks?

    A every day

    B sometimes

    C never

How many cups of coffee do you consume each day?
- **A** two or more
- **B** one or two
- **C** fewer than one

How often do you urinate?
- **A** once or twice a day
- **B** several times a day
- **C** too many times to count

What color is your urine?
- **A** dark yellow
- **B** pale yellow
- **C** clear

If you answered mostly A, you are severely dehydrated, and you drastically need to increase your water intake. If you answered mostly B, you are drinking some water but not enough. Increase your intake to eight glasses each day. If you answered mostly C, you are drinking enough water.

How Healthy Is Your Diet?

If your diet is bad, your body will clog with toxins and not function to its full potential. Here are some common problem areas:

How often do you eat out or get takeout?
- **A** rarely
- **B** occasionally
- **C** most nights

How many servings of vegetables do you eat each day?

- **A** five or more
- **B** one to five
- **C** none

How many servings of fruit do you eat each day?

- **A** three or more
- **B** one to three
- **C** none

How often do you cook your own meals?

- **A** most nights
- **B** occasionally
- **C** rarely

How often do you snack on cookies, chips, and candy?

- **A** rarely
- **B** occasionally
- **C** every day

How often do you crave chocolate?

- **A** rarely
- **B** occasionally
- **C** every day

How often do you eat fish?

- **A** two or three times a week
- **B** once a week
- **C** rarely

How often do you eat fried or fatty foods?

- **A** rarely
- **B** occasionally
- **C** every day

If you answered mostly A, then you are eating well. If you answered mostly B, you are well on the way to healthy eating but could benefit from some changes to your diet. If you answered mostly C, you really would benefit from a dietary overhaul and a detox.

What Sort of Physical State Are You In?

Your current physical state will be one of the key indicators of whether you need to detox.

Are you overweight?

    A no

    B yes

Do you always feel tired?

    A no

    B yes

Do you feel bloated or sick after a meal?

    A no

    B yes

Do you suffer from constipation or diarrhea?

    A no

    B yes

Do you smoke?

    A no

    B yes

Do you drink alcohol to excess or on a daily basis?

    A no

    B yes

Is your blood pressure high?

    A   no

    B   yes

Do you still feel tired when you wake in the morning?

    A   no

    B   yes

Do you regularly exercise at least twice a week?

    A   yes

    B   no

Do you enjoy exercising?

    A   yes

    B   no

If you answered mostly A, you are in good shape and are taking care of your body. If you answered mostly B, you need to start taking better care of your health and would likely benefit from a detox.

How Toxic Is Your Home and Your Life?

Detoxing is not just about changing what you put into your mouth. It also refers to clearing the toxins in your home and personal life. Emotional issues can have a toxic effect on your mental and physical well-being. Chemicals that you use in your home inject physical toxins into your environment that your lungs and your skin absorb.

Do you use three or more cleaning products when cleaning your house?

A yes

B no

Do you use environmentally friendly, chemical-free cleaning products?

A no

B yes

Do you try to buy organic foods whenever possible?

A no

B yes

Does unspoken resentment exist between you and others close to you?

A yes

B no

Are you fighting with any family or friends?

A yes

B no

Are emotional issues affecting your physical health?

A yes

B no

If you answered mostly A, you probably have toxic issues in your environment and personal life. A detox likely could help you clear these issues. If you answered mostly B, you are well on your way to detoxing your emotional and physical environment.

Detox Eating 3

The guidelines for detox eating are quite simple—increase your consumption of detox foods, avoid toxic foods, and increase your water consumption.

Increase Your Intake of Detox Foods

What are detox foods? These are unprocessed foods that are excellent sources of vitamins, minerals, and antioxidants. They are easy to digest and provide plenty of slow-release energy.

Vegetables

Try to eat five servings of vegetables each day in as raw a state as possible. If you must cook them, light steaming maintains the most nutrients. A lot of the nutrients in vegetables are found in or near the skin, so scrub and wash them rather than peel them.

Dark leafy greens, beets, carrots, sweet potatoes, and tomatoes are all high in antioxidants.

Fruit

Fruit is also full of nutrients, essential vitamins, and minerals, and it is high in fiber. Fruit has a high water content and is full of natural sugars, so it is a great food to grab when sugar cravings hit. Try to eat three servings each day.

Grains, Beans, Rice, and Legumes

Grains, beans, rice, and legumes are cheap and nutritious and are full of dietary fiber, nutrients, and vitamins. Try alfalfa, chickpeas, lentils, and pumpkin seeds. Brown rice is preferable to white rice, as it is less refined. While detoxing, avoid barley, oats, rye, and wheat because they all contain gluten, which is difficult to digest (amaranth, buckwheat, corn, millet, quinoa, rice, sorghum, and teff, do not contain gluten).

Seafood

Seafood is a highly nutritious food that is easily digested. Fish (especially the oily varieties, such as salmon, trout, and tuna) is full of omega fatty acids and essential proteins. Although fresh fish is best, canned and frozen varieties are also excellent foods to consume while detoxing.

Yogurt

Although dairy products should be avoided while detoxing, as discussed below, yogurt is one dairy food that is okay to eat. Don't buy artificially sweetened or sugar-laden, fruit-flavored varieties—go for plain, unsweetened types. If you want to sweeten plain yogurt, mix it with honey or some fresh fruit. Acidophilus yogurt helps cleanse your gut of bad bacteria.

Tasty Extras

Herbs and spices, mustard, nuts, oils, olives, seaweed, seeds, tahini, and tofu all add variety and flavor to your diet. Garlic and ginger are especially good for you. Nuts and seeds make an excellent snack food when eaten raw and unsalted.

Chicken and Eggs

While you're doing a short detox, chicken and eggs should be avoided because it takes a while for the body to digest them. However, they are good sources of protein and can be included in your normal healthy eating plan once you have finished the detox. Try to consume free-range eggs whenever possible, as they contain more nutrients, less cholesterol, and fewer toxins, and some people even think they taste better than commercially produced eggs.

Decrease Your Intake of Toxic Foods

What are toxic foods? These are foods that your body takes longer to digest, thus placing extra stress on your organs of elimination and hindering the detox process. They are often processed foods that contain artificial additives and chemicals.

Red Meat

Meat is on the "to avoid" list, because your body has to work extra hard to digest it. It also can contain large quantities of saturated fat, and nonorganic meat may contain traces of growth hormones.

Dairy Products

Dairy products are often high in fat, and lactose can be difficult to digest. Yogurt is the exception to the rule. Unsweetened plain yogurt with acidophilus is permitted when you're detoxing.

Processed Foods and Salt

Processed foods are usually so far removed from their natural states that very little nutritional value remains. These types of foods are laden with fat, sugar, salt, and artificial colors and flavors. Salt causes fluid retention and high blood pressure, so do not add extra salt to your food.

Alcohol and Caffeine

Alcohol and caffeine dehydrate your body and contain toxic substances that your liver has to work overtime to break down.

Gluten

Gluten can be difficult to digest. Such common grains as barley, oats, rye, and wheat all contain gluten. Substitute rice or lentils instead.

Sugar

Sugar is full of empty calories and has an immediate impact on blood-sugar levels, causing them to rise and fall very quickly. Fructose (the natural sugar found in fruit) is fine, but refined white sugar, glucose, and sucrose should all be avoided.

Restaurant and Takeout Foods

Below is a quick cuisine guide to help you choose the healthiest options in restaurants and when you're ordering takeout.

Choosing the Best Foods for Detox

CUISINE	BEST CHOICE (unprocessed, gluten-free, dairy-free, low in salt and sugar)	WORST CHOICE (highly processed, dairy- or meat-based, with gluten, salt, and sugar)
Italian	Fruit-based gelato Grilled fish Salad	Garlic or herb bread (high in fat and gluten) Pasta (high in gluten) Pizza (dairy, gluten, and meat) Risotto (too much butter)
Japanese	Sashimi Steamed rice Sushi	Chicken teriyaki (try to avoid chicken when detoxing)
Indian	Dahl Low-fat yogurt Steamed rice Vegetable or lentil curries	Deep-fried entrées Roti bread (or any other white fried bread) Whole-wheat baked chapati
Asian	Steamed fish with ginger Steamed rice Vegetarian noodle dishes Vegetarian stir-fries with low-sodium soy sauce	Deep-fried entrées Dumplings Meat-based stir-fries Satay sauce
Greek	Greek salad (reduce the amount of or omit the feta cheese)	Baklava Dolmades Moussaka Souvlaki

(cont'd.)

Choosing the Best Foods for Detox (cont'd.)

CUISINE	BEST CHOICE (unprocessed, gluten-free, dairy-free, low in salt and sugar)	WORST CHOICE (highly processed, dairy- or meat-based, with gluten, salt, and sugar)
Seafood	Grilled seafood Salad	Deep-fried seafood French fries
Buffets	Cold seafood Fresh fruit Salad	Breads Cakes Cheesecake Deep-fried appetizers or entrées Mousse Potato salad Rice salad
Burger chains	Fresh fruit Salad Water	Burgers Chicken nuggets Desserts Fries
Sandwich shops	Fresh fruit juices Salad Water	Creamy salads, such as Caesar and potato Sandwiches
Pizza parlors	Salad bar (no potato or creamy dressings) Water	All desserts All pizzas Garlic bread
Fish and chips	Green salad Grilled fish	Deep-fried fish French fries Fried calamari Scalloped potatoes

Drink More Water

The simple rule for water consumption is eight glasses of water each day. Although this may seem like a lot of water if you are not currently drinking it, it really is quite easy to increase your water consumption.

To remember to drink at least six glasses a day, follow this simple plan:

- Drink a glass of water first thing in the morning before you eat or drink anything else.

- Have a glass of water with breakfast, lunch, and dinner.

- Have a glass of water at midmorning and mid-afternoon.

Other ways to help increase your water consumption in order to reach eight glasses a day include the following:

- Keep a jug on the kitchen counter, on the dining-room table, or at your desk at work. Water is easier to drink if it is room temperature.

- Replace caffeinated and alcoholic drinks with water. It is especially important to remember to drink more water when it is hot, when you are exercising, or when you are drinking alcohol to avoid dehydration.

- Always have a glass of water before you exercise, and drink whenever you feel thirsty during exercise.

- Have a glass of water before you start drinking alcohol, and alternate alcoholic drinks with glasses of water. Drink as much water as you can before going to bed.

One of the major benefits of drinking more water is that you actually reduce your hunger levels. People often mistake thirst for hunger and eat when their body really wants water. Water fills you up and helps you eat less.

Detox Living 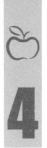 4

"Detox living" refers to making external changes to help your body detox. Exercise, massage, exfoliation, deep breathing, and good posture all help your body eliminate waste, thereby eliminating toxins.

Detoxing your home reduces the amount of chemicals (toxins) that your skin and lungs absorb. Detoxing your emotions reduces the amount of stress on your body, thereby enabling it to function properly and eliminate waste more efficiently.

Exercise

The importance of exercise in detoxing cannot be overstated. The many benefits of exercise include

- faster metabolism
- improved circulation
- better sleep
- increased water consumption
- less constipation

- increased energy level
- improved fitness level
- weight loss
- longer lifespan

You already know that exercise is good for you, but you may find it hard to get motivated or stay motivated when introducing exercise into your lifestyle.

Here are some tips to get you started and keep you on track when the going gets tough:

- **Choose a form of exercise that you enjoy.** Dancing, walking, swimming, playing tennis, and practicing yoga are enjoyable, great forms of exercise.

- **Choose the right type of exercise for your personality.** If you enjoy mixing with other people, chose a social form of exercise, such as an aerobics class, a tennis club, a walking group, or group dance classes. If you need peace and like to exercise on your own, then try yoga or Pilates, exercise DVDs at home, laps in a pool, or quiet early-morning walks.

- **Choose the right time of the day to exercise.** If you are a morning person, get up for an early walk; if you are a night owl, dance the night away.

- **Exercise with a friend.** Having an exercise buddy keeps you motivated and helps remove some of the boredom that comes from repetitious activities. If you can afford it, hire a personal trainer.

Massage

Like exercise, massage offers many benefits, some of which are:

- stress relief
- toned muscles
- relaxation
- improved circulation and lymphatic flow
- lowered blood pressure
- more efficient waste elimination

Massage is easy to do yourself at home. If you have a partner or friend, it is best if you can give each other a massage. Here are some key tips:

- Use the ends of your fingers or the palm of your hand.
- Stroke toward the heart, not away from it (doing so increases venous and lymphatic flow and ensures that no blood is being pushed against closed valves, which might damage blood vessels).
- Make sure the person being massaged is relaxed and comfortable before you start.
- Begin gently before working up to harder strokes.

Exfoliation

Exfoliation rids your body of dry skin cells and helps stimulate your circulatory, lymphatic, and elimination systems. Ideally, you should do it weekly while bathing.

You will need some sort of exfoliating scrub and water. You can buy exfoliating scrubs or make one from salt, sugar, or rolled oats mixed with oil, moisturizer, or honey.

To exfoliate, gently massage yourself all over, and then soak in a warm (not hot) bath. Get out of the bath, leaving the water in, and gently rub in the exfoliating scrub. Get back in the bath to rinse it off. Gently pat yourself dry, and apply moisturizer all over.

Breathing and Posture

Breathing is something you do subconsciously, but you may not realize that there are different ways of breathing. When you are anxious, you take short, sharp, shallow breaths. When you are relaxed, you take longer, deeper, slower breaths, a technique called deep breathing. To practice deep breathing, also known as belly breathing, find a comfortable position either lying on your back or sitting, close your eyes, and place your hand on your belly so you can concentrate on letting your belly rise instead of your chest as you breathe in. Deep breathing causes you to inhale more oxygen, thus relaxing the mind and relieving stress. If you are having trouble taking deep breaths, try breathing in through your nose and exhaling through your mouth. Also, slowly count to five in your head as you breathe in and out.

Good posture is important for detoxing, because it allows your organs to function properly, especially the organs involved with digestion and elimination. To achieve good posture, stick your chest out, place your shoulders back, and hold your head up high. Regularly exercising and sitting erect help maintain good posture.

Meditation

Meditation is one of the best tools for clearing the mind, relaxing the body, and reducing stress. Many meditation recordings are available that will guide you through the process, but it is also easy to meditate on your own by following this exercise:

- Go to a quiet, dark room, and take the phone off the hook or turn off your cell phone.

- Make sure that you are warm and comfortable before you begin the meditation.

- Lie down on a bed or a mat on the floor, and close your eyes.

- Imagine yourself in a relaxing scene, such as lying on a deserted beach and listening to the sound of the waves coming onto shore. Slowly breathe in and out, practicing your deep breathing.

- Starting with your toes and slowly working up your entire body, tense and then relax each part of your body. Feel how heavy and relaxed your limbs are.

- After you have relaxed your entire body, lie still for a few more minutes, listening to the sound of your heavy deep breathing.

- When you are ready to finish the exercise, slowly stretch your limbs and open your eyes.

- Slowly get up and enjoy the feeling of calm that pervades your body.

Detoxing Your Emotions

If you are carrying around old wounds and anger, you are channeling your emotional energy into negative and destructive emotions. These feelings can affect your physical and mental health and drain you of energy.

To detox your emotions, you need to find a way of addressing them so you can move forward and leave the negative emotions behind. This can be a slow and painful process, but it is necessary if you want to grow as a person.

Some ideas for emotional detoxing include:

- Reading self-help books. Many books have been written to help people let go of destructive emotions.

- Writing a letter to the people involved. You don't need to send it—often just the process of writing the letter can make you feel better.

- Seeing a professional counselor. If you have a

long history of issues with family or loved ones, some sessions with a therapist can provide a fresh perspective on your situation and help you move forward.

Sometimes the best way to deal with difficult people is to just accept that they are the way they are and that the only thing you can change is the way you react to them. This realization can be very liberating and allow you to move forward mentally without having to discuss painful issues with these people.

Regardless of the path you take, you will be amazed at how liberated you feel once you are able to let go of anger and old hurts. Detoxifying your emotions has a huge positive effect on your physical and emotional well-being.

Detoxing Your Home

It has never been easier to detox your home. As more people are becoming aware of the need to reduce chemical exposure, the marketplace is responding to this trend by offering green products for sale to consumers. Green alternatives can now be found for myriad applications, including cleaning, doing laundry, washing dishes, etc.

You can also read books or reputable websites to get ideas of how to clean your home using natural products, such as baking soda and vinegar. And don't forget to buy organic products (food and even clothing) as often as possible.

Reducing the amount of chemicals in your home can save you money and helps you rid your environment of the toxins your lungs and skin absorb every day.

Bathrooms

Simple baking soda, lemon juice, and vinegar will clean and sanitize bathroom surfaces. Toilets can be cleaned with white vinegar: Wipe a cloth moistened with vinegar over the toilet's surface, and pour one cup of vinegar down the sides of the bowl and let it soak overnight before flushing the next morning. If the bowl is badly stained, sprinkle baking soda on it and scrub with a brush before pouring vinegar down the sides.

Lemon juice can be used to dissolve soap scum and hard water deposits. Try mixing lemon juice with vinegar or baking soda to make an effective cleaning paste.

Mold can be removed from tile and shower walls with a stiff brush or scouring pad and baking soda. Rinse with water, and then wipe the surface with an old towel or cloth after scrubbing.

Soap scum can be removed by scrubbing with vinegar on a cloth or an old balled-up stocking moistened with warm water. To prevent buildup of mold, wipe down shower walls and the rim of the tub with an old towel after use.

Dusting

Suck up dust with your vacuum or wipe surfaces with an environmentally friendly dusting cloth.

Floors

Wash hard surfaces with a mixture of one cup of vinegar to a half gallon of warm water. Sweep and vacuum regularly to prevent buildup of dust.

Furniture

Mix 1 cup olive oil with ½ cup lemon juice to create a furniture polish perfect for hardwood furniture.

Kitchens

Baking soda will remove most kitchen grime. When dealing with baked-on cooking stains, make a stiff paste of baking soda and water and leave it on the stain for a while before scrubbing it off.

Ceramic tiles can be wiped down with a little white vinegar on a cloth.

Laundry Room

You can use vinegar as a natural fabric softener. This can be especially helpful for families with sensitive skin issues. Add ½ cup of vinegar to the rinse cycle in place of store-bought fabric softener.

5 Detox Plan

This chapter tells you what you need to know to start your own detox program.

Preparing to Detox

Before you start to detox, check with your doctor to ensure that no medical reasons would prohibit you from detoxing.

Do not detox if you are:

- breastfeeding
- pregnant
- suffering from a severe illness

Detoxing Your Pantry

To reduce temptation, clean out and restock your pantry before you start to detox.

Give away or throw out:

- alcohol
- any processed or fast foods, such as cookies, chips, prepared frozen meals, chocolate, and candy

- coffee
- gluten foods, such as wheat, oats, breads, and wheat cereals
- milk, cheese, butter, and other dairy products
- red meat and chicken
- salt and condiments that are high in salt, such as tomato sauce and soy sauce
- sugar

Restock your pantry with:
- beans, nuts, and gluten-free grains
- filtered water
- fresh fish
- fresh herbs, including garlic and ginger
- fruit
- herbal teas
- olive oil
- rice (brown rice is preferable due to its added nutritional value)
- soy milk
- unsweetened natural yogurt with acidophilus
- vegetables

Detoxing at Home

Once you have acquired your dietary requirements, add the following to your detox kit:

- an aromatherapy burner and oils
- exfoliating cream
- a loofah
- massage oils
- moisturizer

The Seven-Day Detox Plan

Detoxing is easy—just follow the guidelines below.

The Week Before

Make your life easier by making some changes to your diet in the week before the detox. Cut down on caffeine, replace alcohol and soft drinks with water, and increase your water consumption to eight glasses of water a day.

Day 1

Start the day with a full body massage and exfoliation. After your morning glass of water, make a fresh fruit and vegetable juice. Then follow the eating and living guidelines below.

Days 1 Through 7

Every day try to do the following things:

- Drink eight glasses of water.
- Start each day with a fresh juice made with fruit and vegetables.
- Eat one serving of rice (brown rice is preferable due to its added nutritional value).
- Eat five servings of vegetables.

- Eat two servings of fruit.
- Eat at least three meals.
- Eat one serving of unsweetened, plain yogurt with acidophilus.
- Eat two servings of grains, beans, or fish.
- Exercise for thirty minutes.
- Concentrate on your posture.
- Practice deep breathing for ten minutes.
- Sleep for at least eight hours each night.

Day 7

End the week with another full body massage and exfoliation. Spend some time relaxing and meditating, and savor the freshness of the food you are eating.

Side Effects

When you start to detox, you may experience some side effects as your body rids itself of the toxins that have built up inside, such as headaches, skin problems, lethargy, a change in bowel movements, or unusual body odor. These side effects will pass, and by the end of the week you should feel revitalized and energized.

Living the Detox Way

After your detox week, you can continue to reap the benefits of the *Pocket Detox* without having to follow the strict seven-day plan. You can reintroduce dairy, cheese, eggs, chicken, and wheat products into your diet, but try to avoid reintroducing caffeine, alcohol, and processed foods on a regular basis.

Some overall changes to your diet and lifestyle can include:

- drinking eight glasses of water a day
- exercising at least three times a week
- replacing coffee with herbal tea
- exfoliating once a week
- eating four servings of vegetables and three servings of fruit each day
- choosing unprocessed foods
- meditating once a week
- eating as wide a variety of foods as possible

If you incorporate these changes into your life, you will find you feel better and have a lot more energy. If you feel yourself slipping back into bad eating habits and forgetting to exercise, you can recharge your body by doing another seven-day detox. How you use the plan is your choice—just remember that your body is a machine that can only function according to what you put inside it.

If you want to increase your energy levels and take control of your life, *Pocket Detox* provides you with all the tools you need for success.

Your Detox Choices by Food Category

6

The detox tables come in two different arrangements for ease of use. The first table is grouped by food categories (e.g., breads, fruits, dairy). This allows you to immediately see the least-toxic choice for a particular type of food and helps you avoid the most toxic choices. The second table, which is in Chapter 7, is an alphabetical listing of foods (e.g., banana, rice, lentils) designed to serve as a quick reference when you already know exactly what type of food you are looking for.

These tables cover the most common food categories and do not cover most specific food brands or fast foods. This is because specific, prepared name brands and fast foods are generally processed foods, which are not suitable for detoxing. The food values in these tables refer to fresh produce and foods suitable for detoxing. When a reference is made to processed foods, it is a general reference to that type of processed food, because there is no real difference between brands. For example, all types of cookies, regardless of brand, are to be avoided when detoxing.

The table includes three categories for the foods:

- **detox foods**—These are foods that you can enjoy while detoxing and should form the main basis of your normal diet.

- **foods to eat in moderation**—These should be not be consumed while you are doing the seven-day detox, but they can be enjoyed in moderation as part of your regular diet.

- **toxic foods**—These are absolute no-nos while detoxing and are best avoided altogether or eaten very rarely in the course of your normal diet.

✓ Detox Choice	⊖ Eat in Moderation	✗ Toxic Choice
BEANS AND LEGUMES		
Alfalfa sprouts	Baked beans	Refried beans
Black beans	Canned beans	
Borlotti beans		
Butter beans		
Chickpeas		
Dried beans		
Green beans		
Kidney beans		
Lentils		
Lima beans		
Mung beans		
Navy beans		
Snake beans		
Soya beans		
Split peas		
String beans		

(cont'd.)

✓ Detox Choice	⊖ Eat in Moderation	✕ Toxic Choice
BEVERAGES		
Fruit juice, freshly squeezed, no added sugar Fruit and vegetable juice, freshly squeezed, no added sugar Coffee Herbal tea, no sugar or milk Vegetable juice, freshly squeezed Water, bottled Water, filtered Water, tap	Black tea Fruit juice, sweetened Soda water Tonic water	Alcohol (beer, wine, spirits) Caffeinated soft drinks (Coke, Pepsi, Red Bull) Soft drinks, naturally or artificially sweetened Sport drinks
COOKIES, CRACKERS, CAKES, AND PASTRIES		
No cookie, cake, or pastry forms part of the detox diet	Pancakes Rice crackers, plain Sponge cake, unfrosted and without whipped cream Water crackers	Cakes, all types except sponge Chocolate cookies Cream-filled cookies, such as Oreos Savory crackers Shortbread Sweet rolls
BREADS		
Gluten should be avoided while detoxing. This rules out most breads.	Brown bread Gluten-free bread (from health-food store or super-market) Multigrain bread Pumpernickel bread	Croissants Donuts Hot dog buns Melba toast Sliced white bread White bread rolls

(cont'd.)

✓ Detox Choice	⊖ Eat in Moderation	✗ Toxic Choice

BREADS (cont'd.)

| | Rye bread
Sourdough bread
Soy and linseed
   bread | |

BREAKFAST CEREALS

| No breakfast cereal is suitable for detox, because they are all high in gluten, salt, or sugar. | All Bran
Plain muesli
Oats
Shredded wheat products, such as Mini Wheats
Raisin Bran
Shredded Wheat
Special K | Any breakfast cereal with added sugar
Cocoa Puffs
Corn Flakes
Crispix
Froot Loops
Rice Krispies |

CEREALS, RICE, AND GRAINS

| Arborio rice
Basmati rice
Brown rice
Calrose rice
Jasmine rice
Long-grain rice
Quinoa
Short-grain rice | Barley
Buckwheat
Couscous
Cracked wheat (bulgar)
Linseed | |

CONDIMENTS AND SEASONINGS

| Chilis
Garlic
Herbs
Hummus
Lemon juice
Lime juice
Mustard
Pepper | Mayonnaise
Soy sauce, low-sodium
Tartar sauce
Tomato sauce
Teriyaki sauce
Worcestershire sauce | Salt |

(cont'd.)

✔ **Detox Choice**	⊖ **Eat in Moderation**	✖ **Toxic Choice**
CONDIMENTS AND SEASONINGS (cont'd.)		
Spices Tamari Tzatziki		
DAIRY		

Acidophilus yogurt,
   unsweetened
Rice milk
Soy milk
	Cheese, reduced fat
	Gelato, fruit based
	Ice cream, low fat,
	   fruit based
	Milk, reduced fat
	Milk, skim
		Butter
		Cheese, full fat
		Condensed milk
		Custard
		Ice cream, full fat
		Milk, full fat

FATS, NUTS, AND OILS		

Almonds, unsalted
Brazil nuts, unsalted
Cashews, unsalted
Hazelnuts
Macadamia nuts,
   unsalted
Olive oil
Peanuts, unsalted
Pecans
Pinenuts
Polyunsaturated fats
Pumpkin seeds
Sesame seeds
Sunflower seeds
Walnuts
	Almonds, salted
	Brazil nuts, salted
	Cashews, salted
	Macadamia nuts,
	   salted
	Mixed nuts, salted
	Peanuts, salted
		Butter and other
		   high-fat dairy
		   products
		Meat fat (e.g., bacon
		   fat, lard)
		Crisco/shortening

FRUIT		
Apples Apricots Avocados Bananas	Canned fruit	

(cont'd.)

✓ Detox Choice	− Eat in Moderation	✗ Toxic Choice
FRUIT (cont'd.)		
Blackberries		
Blueberries		
Cantaloupes		
Cherries		
Cranberries		
Dried fruit		
Figs		
Grapefruits		
Grapes		
Honeydew melons		
Kiwis		
Lemons		
Limes		
Lychees		
Mandarins		
Mangoes		
Nectarines		
Oranges		
Papayas		
Peaches		
Pineapples		
Pears		
Plums		
Prunes		
Raspberries		
Rhubarb		
Strawberries		
Tomatoes		
Watermelons		
MEAT AND POULTRY		
Meat and poultry are best avoided during detox.	Beef, lean Chicken, lean Duck, lean	Bacon Chicken nuggets Fatty meat

(cont'd.)

Detox Choice	Eat in Moderation	Toxic Choice

MEAT AND POULTRY (cont'd.)

Meat and poultry are best avoided during detox.	Eggs Ham, lean, off the bone Lamb, lean Ground beef, lean Pork, lean Veal Venison	Hot dogs Ground beef, high fat Processed meats and cold cuts

NOODLES

Fresh rice noodles Glass noodles Mung bean (cellophane) noodles Vermicelli	Egg noodles Hokkien noodles Wheat noodles	Ramen noodles

PASTA

Gluten-free pasta Rice pasta	Capellini Fettuccini Gnocchi Linguini Macaroni Penne Rigatoni Shell pasta Spaghetti Whole-grain pasta	Canned pasta Filled pasta Lasagna Macaroni and cheese Ravioli

SEAFOOD

Fish, all types Sashimi Sushi	Clams Crab Lobster	Anchovies

(cont'd.)

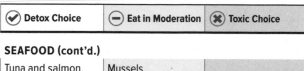

✓ Detox Choice	⊖ Eat in Moderation	✖ Toxic Choice
SEAFOOD (cont'd.)		
Tuna and salmon, fresh or canned	Mussels Oysters Prawns Scallops Smoked oysters and mussels Smoked salmon and trout Squid	
SNACK FOODS		
Almonds, unsalted Brazil nuts, unsalted Cashews, unsalted Fruit, fresh or dried Hazelnuts Macadamia nuts, unsalted Peanuts, unsalted Pecans Pinenuts Popcorn, unsalted and unbuttered Pumpkin seeds Sesame seeds Sunflower seeds Vegetable sticks Walnuts	Almonds, salted Brazil nuts, salted Canned fruit Cashews, salted Macadamia nuts, salted Mixed nuts, salted Peanuts, salted	Candy Cheese puffs (such as Cheetos) Chocolate Corn chips Donuts French fries Fruit snacks and leathers (roll-ups) Muesli bars Potato chips Processed foods Salty snacks

(cont'd.)

⊘ Detox Choice	⊖ Eat in Moderation	⊗ Toxic Choice
SOUP		
Lentil soup, home-made Tomato soup, home-made Vegetable soup, homemade	Chicken soup, home-made Consommé Split-pea soup, homemade	Canned soup Chicken noodle soup, commercial Packet soups
SPREADS, SUGARS, AND SWEETENERS		
Hummus, homemade Honey Maple syrup Peanut butter, home-made, unsalted Tahini	Golden syrup Jam, commercial Jam, homemade Peanut butter, commercial	Nutella Sugar (white and brown)
VEGETABLES		
Alfalfa Artichokes Asparagus Bean sprouts Beets Broccoli Corn Carrots Cabbage Cauliflower Celery Cucumbers Eggplant Fennel Frozen vegetables Green beans Leeks	Canned vegetables	

(cont'd.)

⊘ **Detox Choice**	⊖ **Eat in Moderation**	⊗ **Toxic Choice**

VEGETABLES (cont'd.)

Lettuce		
Mushrooms		
Onions		
Parsnips		
Potatoes		
Pumpkins		
Sweet potatoes		
Turnips		

Your Detox Food Choices in Alphabetical Order 7

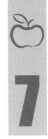

The table in this chapter is simply an alphabetical listing of common foods (e.g., banana, rice, lentils). It is designed to serve as a quick reference when you already know what type of food you are looking for but want to find out if it is highly compatible with your detox diet, should be eaten in moderation, or should be avoided completely.

The table covers the most common food categories and does not cover most specific food brands or fast foods.

Quick Detox Ratings of Foods in Alphabetical Order

Food	Detox Choice	Eat in Moderation	Toxic Choice
Acidophilus yogurt, unsweetened	✅		
Alcohol (beer, wine, spirits)			✖
Alfalfa sprouts	✅		
All bran			
Almonds, salted		➖	
Almonds, unsalted	✅		

(cont'd.)

Food	Detox Choice	Eat in Moderation	Toxic Choice
Anchovies			✖
Apples	✔		
Apricots	✔		
Arborio rice	✔		
Artichokes	✔		
Asparagus	✔		
Avocados	✔		
Bacon			✖
Bananas	✔		
Barley		⊖	
Basmati rice	✔		
Bean sprouts	✔		
Beans, borlotti	✔		
Beans, butter	✔		
Beans, dried	✔		
Beans, green	✔		
Beans, kidney	✔		
Beans, lima	✔		
Beans, mung	✔		
Beans, navy	✔		
Beans, refried			✖
Beans, snake	✔		
Beans, soya	✔		

(cont'd.)

Food	Detox Choice	Eat in Moderation	Toxic Choice
Beans, string	✓		
Beef, lean		⊖	
Beer			✗
Beets	✓		
Black beans	✓		
Blackberries	✓		
Blueberries	✓		
Borlotti beans	✓		
Brazil nuts, salted		⊖	
Brazil nuts, unsalted	✓		
Bread rolls, white			✗
Bread, brown		⊖	
Bread, gluten free		⊖	
Bread, linseed		⊖	
Bread, pumpernickel		⊖	
Bread, rye		⊖	
Bread, sourdough		⊖	
Bread, soy and linseed		⊖	
Bread, white			✗
Breakfast cereal with added sugar			✗
Broccoli	✓		
Brown bread		⊖	

(cont'd.)

Food	Detox Choice	Eat in Moderation	Toxic Choice
Brown rice	✅		
Buckwheat		⊖	
Butter			✖
Butter beans	✅		
Cabbage	✅		
Caffeinated soft drinks (Coke, Pepsi, Red Bull)			✖
Cake, sponge, unfrosted and without whipped cream		⊖	
Cakes, all types except sponge			✖
Calrose rice	✅		
Candy			✖
Canned fruit		⊖	
Canned pasta			✖
Canned soups			✖
Canned vegetables		⊖	
Cantaloupes	✅		
Capellini		⊖	
Carrots	✅		
Cashews, salted		⊖	
Cashews, unsalted	✅		
Cauliflower	✅		
Celery	✅		

(cont'd.)

Food	Detox Choice	Eat in Moderation	Toxic Choice
Cellophane noodles	✓		
Cereal, breakfast with added sugar			✗
Cheese, full fat			✗
Cheese puffs (such as Cheese Doodles or Cheetos)			✗
Cheese, reduced fat		⊖	
Cherries	✓		
Chicken noodle soup, commercial			✗
Chicken nuggets			✗
Chicken soup, homemade		⊖	
Chicken, lean		⊖	
Chickpeas	✓		
Chilies	✓		
Chips, corn			✗
Chips, hot			✗
Chips, potato			✗
Chocolate			✗
Clams		⊖	
Cocoa Puffs			✗
Coffee			✗
Condensed milk			✗
Consommé		⊖	

(cont'd.)

Food	Detox Choice	Eat in Moderation	Toxic Choice
Cookies, chocolate			✖
Cookies, cream-filled (such as Oreos)			✖
Corn	✔		
Corn chips			✖
Cornflakes			✖
Couscous		⊖	
Crab		⊖	
Cracked wheat (bulgar)		⊖	
Crackers, plain rice		⊖	
Crackers, savory			✖
Crackers, sweet			✖
Crackers, water		⊖	
Cranberries	✔		
Crisco			✖
Crispix			✖
Croissants			✖
Cucumber	✔		
Custard			✖
Dairy products, high fat			✖
Donuts			✖
Dried beans	✔		
Dried fruit	✔		

(cont'd.)

Food	Detox Choice	Eat in Moderation	Toxic Choice
Duck, lean		⊖	
Egg noodles		⊖	
Eggplant	✓		
Eggs		⊖	
Fatty meat			✗
Fennel	✓		
Fettuccini		⊖	
Figs	✓		
Filled pasta			✗
Fish, all types	✓		
Fresh fruit	✓		
Fresh rice noodles	✓		
Froot Loops			✗
Frozen vegetables	✓		
Fruit and vegetable juice, freshly squeezed, no added sugar	✓		
Fruit-based gelato		⊖	
Fruit juice, freshly squeezed, no added sugar	✓		
Fruit juice, sweetened		⊖	
Fruit, canned		⊖	
Fruit, fresh or dried	✓		
Fruit leather (e.g., Fruit Roll Ups)			✗

(cont'd.)

Food	Detox Choice	Eat in Moderation	Toxic Choice
Full-fat cheese			✖
Garlic	✔		
Gelato, fruit based		⊖	
Glass noodles	✔		
Gluten-free bread		⊖	
Gluten-free pasta	✔		
Gnocchi		⊖	
Golden syrup		⊖	
Grapefruit	✔		
Grapes	✔		
Green beans	✔		
Ground beef, high fat			✖
Ground beef, lean		⊖	
Ham, lean, off the bone		⊖	
Hazelnuts	✔		
Herbal tea, no sugar or milk	✔		
Herbs	✔		
Hokkien noodles		⊖	
Hummus, homemade	✔		
Honey	✔		
Honeydew melon	✔		
French fries			✖
Hot dog buns			✖

(cont'd.)

Food	Detox Choice	Eat in Moderation	Toxic Choice
Hot dogs			⊗
Ice cream, full fat			⊗
Ice cream, low fat, fruit based		⊖	
Jam, commercial		⊖	
Jam, homemade		⊖	
Jasmine rice	✓		
Juice, fruit and vegetable, freshly squeezed, no added sugar	✓		
Juice, fruit, freshly squeezed, no added sugar	✓		
Kidney beans	✓		
Kiwis	✓		
Lamb, lean		⊖	
Lard			⊗
Lasagna			⊗
Leeks	✓		
Lemon juice	✓		
Lemons	✓		
Lentil soup, homemade	✓		
Lentils	✓		
Lettuce	✓		
Lima beans	✓		
Lime juice	✓		

(cont'd.)

Food	Detox Choice	Eat in Moderation	Toxic Choice
Limes	✓		
Linguini		⊖	
Linseed bread		⊖	
Liquor			✗
Lobster		⊖	
Long-grain rice	✓		
Lychees	✓		
Macadamia nuts, salted		⊖	
Macadamia nuts, unsalted	✓		
Macaroni		⊖	
Macaroni and cheese			✗
Mandarins	✓		
Mango	✓		
Maple syrup	✓		
Mayonnaise		⊖	
Meat fat (i.e., the fat on a cut of meat)			✗
Meat, fatty			✗
Meat, processed			✗
Melba toast			✗
Milk, condensed			✗
Milk, full fat		⊖	
Milk, reduced fat		⊖	

(cont'd.)

Food	Detox Choice	Eat in Moderation	Toxic Choice
Milk, rice	✅		
Milk, skim		⊖	
Milk, soy	✅		
Mini Wheats		⊖	
Muesli bars			✖
Muesli, plain		⊖	
Mung bean (cellophane) noodles	✅		
Mung beans	✅		
Mushrooms	✅		
Mussels		⊖	
Mustard	✅		
Navy beans	✅		
Nectarines	✅		
Noodles, cellophane	✅		
Noodles, egg		⊖	
Noodles, fresh rice	✅		
Noodles, glass	✅		
Noodles, hokkien		⊖	
Noodles, ramen			✖
Noodles, wheat		⊖	
Nutella			✖
Nutrigrain			✖
Nuts, salted, mixed		⊖	

(cont'd.)

Food	Detox Choice	Eat in Moderation	Toxic Choice
Oats		⊖	
Olive oil	✓		
Onions	✓		
Oranges	✓		
Oreos			✕
Oysters		⊖	
Oysters and mussels, smoked		⊖	
Parsnips	✓		
Pasta, canned			✕
Pasta, filled			✕
Pasta, gluten free			
Pasta, rice	✓		
Pasta, shell		⊖	
Pasta, whole grain		⊖	
Papayas	✓		
Peaches	✓		
Peanut butter, homemade, unsalted	✓		
Peanut butter, commercial		⊖	
Peanuts, salted		⊖	
Peanuts, unsalted	✓		
Pears	✓		
Pecans	✓		

(cont'd.)

Food	Detox Choice	Eat in Moderation	Toxic Choice
Penne		⊖	
Pepper	✓		
Pineapple	✓		
Pinenuts	✓		
Plums	✓		
Polyunsaturated fats (e.g., vegetable oil, mayonnaise)	✓		
Popcorn, unsalted and unbuttered	✓		
Pork, lean		⊖	
Potatoes	✓		
Potato chips			✗
Potatoes, sweet	✓		
Prawns		⊖	
Processed foods			✗
Processed meats			✗
Prunes	✓		
Pumpernickel bread		⊖	
Pumpkin	✓		
Pumpkin seeds	✓		
Quinoa	✓		
Raisin Bran		⊖	
Raspberries	✓		

(cont'd.)

Food	Detox Choice	Eat in Moderation	Toxic Choice
Ravioli			⊗
Reduced-fat cheese		⊖	
Refried beans			⊗
Rhubarb	✓		
Rice, arborio	✓		
Rice, basmati	✓		
Rice, brown	✓		
Rice, calrose	✓		
Rice, jasmine	✓		
Rice, long grain	✓		
Rice, short grain	✓		
Rice Krispies			⊗
Rice crackers, plain		⊖	
Rice milk	✓		
Rice pasta	✓		
Rigatoni		⊖	
Rye bread		⊖	
Salami			⊗
Salmon and trout, smoked		⊖	
Salmon, fresh or canned	✓		
Salt			⊗
Salted mixed nuts		⊖	
Salty snacks			⊗

(cont'd.)

Food	Detox Choice	Eat in Moderation	Toxic Choice
Sandwich cookies, cream-filled (such as Oreos)			✖
Sashimi	✔		
Sauce, tartar		⊖	
Sauce, teriyaki		⊖	
Sauce, tomato		⊖	
Sauce, Worcestershire		⊖	
Savory crackers			✖
Scallops		⊖	
Seeds, pumpkin	✔		
Seeds, sesame	✔		
Seeds, sunflower	✔		
Sesame seeds	✔		
Shell pasta		⊖	
Short-grain rice	✔		
Shortbread			✖
Smoked oysters and mussels		⊖	
Smoked salmon and trout		⊖	
Snacks, salty			✖
Snake beans	✔		
Soda water		⊖	
Soft drinks, caffeinated (Coke, Pepsi, Red Bull)			✖

(cont'd.)

Food	Detox Choice	Eat in Moderation	Toxic Choice
Soft drinks, naturally or artificially sweetened			⊗
Soup, canned			⊗
Soup, chicken noodle, commercial			⊗
Soup, homemade chicken		⊖	
Soup, homemade split pea		⊖	
Soup, lentil, homemade	✓		
Soup, packet			⊗
Sourdough bread		⊖	
Soy and linseed bread		⊖	
Soy milk	✓		
Soy sauce, low sodium		⊖	
Soya beans	✓		
Spaghetti		⊖	
Special K		⊖	
Spices	✓		
Spirits			⊗
Split-pea soup, homemade		⊖	
Split peas	✓		
Sponge cake, unfrosted and without whipped cream		⊖	
Sport drinks			⊗
Sprouts, bean	✓		

(cont'd.)

Food	Detox Choice	Eat in Moderation	Toxic Choice
Squid		⊖	
Strawberries	✓		
String beans	✓		
Sugar			✗
Sunflower seeds	✓		
Sushi	✓		
Sweet crackers			✗
Sweet potato	✓		
Sweetened fruit juice		⊖	
Sweets			✗
Tahini	✓		
Tamari	✓		
Tartar sauce		⊖	
Tea, black		⊖	
Tea, herbal, no sugar or milk	✓		
Teriyaki sauce		⊖	
Toast, melba			✗
Tomato sauce		⊖	
Tomato soup, homemade	✓		
Tomatoes	✓		
Tonic water		⊖	
Trans fat (shortening, such as Crisco)			✗

(cont'd.)

Food	Detox Choice	Eat in Moderation	Toxic Choice
Tuna and salmon, fresh or canned	✓		
Turnips	✓		
Tzatziki	✓		
Veal		⊖	
Vegetable juice, freshly squeezed	✓		
Vegetable soup, homemade	✓		
Vegetable sticks	✓		
Vegetables, canned		⊖	
Vegetables, frozen	✓		
Venison		⊖	
Vermicelli	✓		
Walnuts	✓		
Water crackers		⊖	
Water, bottled	✓		
Water, filtered	✓		
Water, soda		⊖	
Water, tap	✓		
Water, tonic		⊖	
Watermelon	✓		
Wheat noodles		⊖	
Wheat products, shredded, such as Mini Wheats		⊖	

(cont'd.)

Food	Detox Choice	Eat in Moderation	Toxic Choice
White bread			⊗
White bread rolls			⊗
Whole-grain pasta		⊖	
Wine			⊗
Worcestershire sauce		⊖	
Yogurt, acidophilus, unsweetened	✓		

Resources

Websites

www.ewg.org
Includes "Dirty Dozen" and "Clean Fifteen" lists that note which produce must absolutely be organic to avoid increased exposure to pesticides and which produce is probably safe even when conventionally grown.

www.livestrong.com
Includes food and fitness trackers, a smoking cessation plan, healthy recipes, and detox product reviews.

www.elsonhaas.com
Provides health and wellness information, tips, and advice from Elson M. Haas, MD, author of several detox books, and his team of health and medical professionals.

www.healthy.net
Provides health news, information on nutrition, and recipes.

http://altmedicine.about.com
Includes many articles on the subject of detoxing.

www.mindbodygreen.com
Includes articles on detoxing your home as well as on the many ways to detox your body.

Books

Bennett, Peter, Sara Faye, and Stephen Barrie. *7-Day Detox Miracle*. Rocklin, CA: Prima Health, 2001.

DeJong, Michael. *Clean: The Humble Art of Zen-Cleansing.* New York: Sterling/Joost Elffers, 2007.

Haas, Elson, and Daniella Chace. *The New Detox Diet: The Complete Guide for Lifelong Vitality with Recipes, Menus, and Detox Plans.* New York: Random House, 2004.

Harper, Jennifer. *Detox Handbook*. London: DK Adult, 2002.

Junger, Alejandro. *Clean — Expanded Edition: The Revolutionary Program to Restore the Body's Natural Ability to Heal Itself.* New York: HarperOne, 2012.

Niemerow, Adina. *Super Cleanse Revised Edition: Detox Your Body for Long-Lasting Health and Beauty.* New York: William Morrow, 2011.

Page, Linda. *Detoxification: All You Need to Know to Recharge, Renew and Rejuvenate Your Body, Mind and Spirit.* Carmel Valley, CA: Traditional Wisdom, Inc., 2002.

Shazzie, and David Wolfe. *Detox Your World: Quick and Lasting Results for a Beautiful Mind, Body, and Spirit*. Berkeley, CA: North Atlantic Books, 2012.

Snyder, Kimberly. *The Beauty Detox Solution: Eat Your Way to Radiant Skin, Renewed Energy and the Body You've Always Wanted*. Buffalo, NY: Harlequin, 2011.

Wootan, Gerald Don, and Matthew Brittain Phillips. *Detox Diets For Dummies*. Hoboken, NJ: For Dummies (Wiley), 2010.

Zurich, Linda. *Detoxification: 70 Ways To Cleanse, Clear & Purify Your Body, Space & Life*. Linda J. Zurich, 2011.